DAISY EVERLEY

SUPER IMMUNITY

The Ultimate Guide to Immune Food Solutions, Learn All About the Food and Diet That Can Boost Your Immune System for Good Health and Long Life

Descrierea CIP a Bibliotecii Naţionale a României
DAISY EVERLEY
    SUPER IMMUNITY. The Ultimate Guide to Immune Food Solutions, Learn All About the Food and Diet That Can Boost Your Immune System for Good Health and Long Life / Daisy Everley – Bucharest: Editura My Ebook, 2020
    ISBN

DAISY EVERLEY

SUPER IMMUNITY

The Ultimate Guide to Immune Food Solutions, Learn All About the Food and Diet That Can Boost Your Immune System for Good Health and Long Life

My Ebook Publishing House
Bucharest, 2020

TABLE OF CONTENTS

INTRODUCTION

All of us are aware of how important it is to eat a healthy diet when it comes to maintaining and supporting your overall health and well-being. However, it's all too easy to overlook the role that food can play in boosting our immune systems and helping us to withstand diseases and illnesses.

We all know that if we eat plenty of fruits and vegetables, as well as foods with a high content of vitamins and minerals, we can ensure a better quality of life, with less risk of becoming unwell due to malnutrition or obesity. Yet, all too often, we don't realize that we need to eat the right kinds of food to keep our immunity levels high.

Without an adequate, healthy diet, we can begin to become unwell and suffer from a host of medical issues. In this book, therefore, we look at which foods we should be eating for optimal immunity, and how those foods can help our bodies to combat disease. We also look at ways of combining those foods to create the ultimate immunity-boosting diet for a longer and healthier life.

Read on to discover more about what you should be adding to your daily diet and the different benefits that those foods could be bringing to your health and well-being. With the advice contained in this book, you should find that it's easier than you imagined to create the best possible diet to boost your immunity and give you the optimal resilience to disease and sickness.

CHAPTER 1

THE IMMUNITY PROBLEM – AN OVERVIEW

Your immune system has a key role to play in your body, keeping you safe from the micro-organisms that can cause diseases. If germs successfully invade your body, you can become sick. So, finding ways to intervene in this process and give your immunity a boost couldn't be more important.

Without a strong immune system, the result is a disease. While some of the illnesses, such as the common cold, may be mild and easily overcome, others can be much more serious and even life- threatening. So, how is it possible to improve your immunity?

The concept of giving your immune system a boost is an enticing one, however for generations, finding ways to do it has proved to be elusive. This is because your immune system isn't a single entity – it's an entire system that requires harmony and balance to function effectively. Even today, researchers still lack knowledge about how the immune response interconnects, and no direct links have been scientifically proven between enhanced immune function and lifestyle.

Nevertheless, that doesn't mean that the effect of your lifestyle on your immunity isn't intriguing. Researchers have been exploring the effect of a number of factors on immune responses in humans and recommend that the best line of defense when it comes to your immunity is choosing a healthy diet. This will naturally keep your immune system as strong as possible.

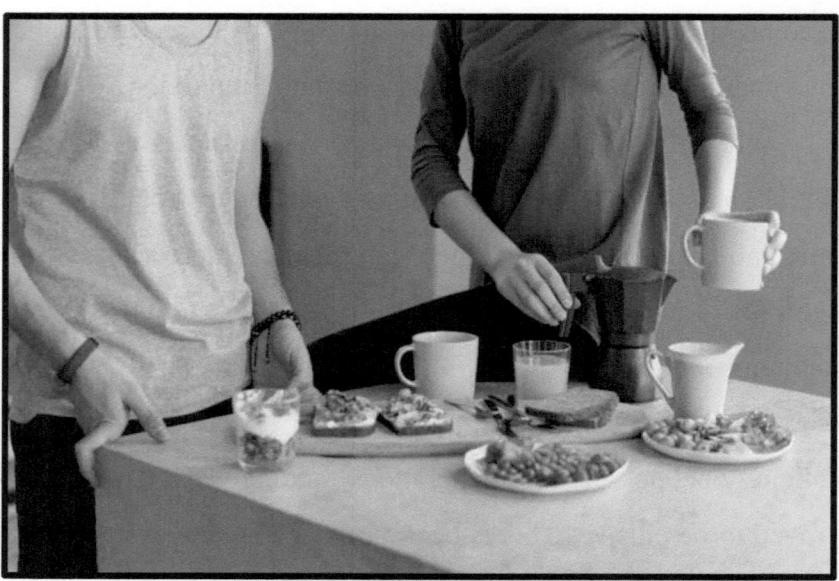

How Does the Immune System Work?

Your immune system is your body's defense from infection, attacking germs and keeping you healthy.

The immune system contains leukocytes or white blood cells, which have a vital part to play in destroying invading organisms. Whenever foreign substances known as antigens are sensed by your body, your immune system works hard to recognize them and eradicate them.

When your immune system is strong, it can identify these potential threats quickly and eliminate them rapidly before they have a chance to make you unwell. However, if your immunity is compromised for any reason, you're at risk of becoming ill and suffering from a disease caused by the antigens your body has been invaded by.

What Affects the Immune System?

There are a number of factors that affect the immune system. These include:

Stress – if you're subjected to prolonged episodes of intense stress, your immunity is impacted. Stress increases cortisol production in the brain. This impairs the way that the T-cells that fight infection work.

Loneliness – if you're lonely, your immunity can be impaired. The increased anxiety that is caused by loneliness suppresses the immune system.

Living a sedentary lifestyle – if you sit for too long and avoid exercise, your body struggles to combat infections.

Excessive exercise – while a sedentary life affects your immune system, so does extreme exercise. Overtraining syndrome is debilitating and makes your body more vulnerable to diseases.

Nicotine – exposure to nicotine, either through regular cigarettes or vaping can harm your immunity. This is due to the increased cortisol levels that nicotine creates paired with a reduction in the formation of B cell antibodies.

UV radiation – harmful ultraviolet rays can weaken your immune system, affecting the cells that trigger immune responses and lowering your defenses.

Diet – if you eat unhealthy foods like saturated fats, sugar and salt, you are at risk of obesity. This impacts your immunity by reducing the function and number of white blood cells required to fight infections.

Alcohol – excessive alcohol consumption reduces your immune response to any invading pathogens. Acetaldehyde, the major metabolite in alcohol, impairs the lungs' ciliary function so they become more susceptible to viral and bacterial invasion. Alcohol also negatively affects the body's process of breaking down and attacking viruses and bacteria increasing the risk of infection.

Grief – a tragic event may weaken your immune response by boosting the hormones and nerve chemicals that put you at a greater risk of viral infections. Bereavement has been linked with immune imbalances and increased cortisol response.

Ways of Boosting Your Immunity

Modern medicine has acknowledged that the body and mind have a strong link. Many maladies have been linked to emotional stress, and stress has been shown to negatively impact immune function. Therefore, one way to improve your immunity is to try to limit the stress in your life. Practice mindfulness and stress reduction techniques such as yoga or meditation to help increase your resistance to disease. Taking regular moderate exercise will also help to naturally give your immunity a boost.

Your immune system requires regular, good nourishment to function properly. It has long been known by scientists that those who are malnourished have a greater vulnerability to infections.

Deficiencies in micronutrients like selenium, zinc, folic acid, iron, and vitamins E, B6, C, and A can alter your immune response. Therefore, ensuring you consume enough of these nutrients is imperative to boosting your immunity.

It's possible to buy supplements that can support your immunity but it's best to try to achieve this by eating a healthier diet.

Immunity and Your Age

Most of us are aware that, as we get older, we experience more diseases and are more at risk from any viruses that are out there. However, we don't always recognize why this is the case.

When we get older, we experience a reduced immune response and this, in turn, leads to more infections and illnesses.

Although some people get older and remain healthy, the elderly have been shown to be more at risk of infectious diseases. In older people, a connection has been shown between immunity and nutrition. Older people often eat less food, in general, and have a less varied diet.

This can lead to micronutrient malnutrition which is known to reduce immunity. It's therefore imperative for the elderly to ensure a healthy, balanced diet to protect themselves from illnesses. With a diet that is rich in vitamins, minerals, and other important nutrients, it's possible to enjoy a healthy lifestyle right through your later years.

CHAPTER 2

NUTRITION FOR YOUR IMMUNE SYSTEM

We've all heard the saying "you are what you eat". This is especially true when it comes to your immune system. Research has shown that if you eat well, your immune system will benefit.

Your immune system needs good nutrition to function properly, and if you're malnourished, deficient in micronutrients, or don't get enough of the right kinds of food to keep you healthy, not only will your overall well-being suffer but your immunity will take a nosedive too. People who eat a poor-quality diet are unable to maintain a healthy immune system. As a result, they have a greater chance of developing ongoing health issues as well as short-term illnesses.

You are not only putting yourself at risk of coughs, colds, flu, and other relatively minor conditions, but you're also more likely to develop more serious medical problems like diabetes, hypertension or cancer. Therefore, knowing the link between nutrition and immunity is imperative so that you can take action to improve your diet and, therefore, your overall well-being.

Malnourishment and its Role in low Immunity

If your body isn't receiving enough nutrition, the number of white blood cells decreases, and this makes it hard to fight illnesses and heal diseases.

When you are experiencing malnutrition, your body cannot recover fully as wounds require protein, energy, minerals, and vitamins to fully heal. Also, if you're malnourished you are at a higher risk of cancer and will struggle to tolerate the chemotherapy necessary to treat it. Of course, if you're malnourished you will also be at a higher risk of infections and illnesses.

While we tend to think of malnourishment as something that only occurs in developing countries, in fact, there are surprising numbers of people in the USA and other developed nations who are malnourished due to a lack of appropriate nutrients in their diet. While they may physically eat sufficient food, unfortunately, they don't choose the right foods to give them the nutrition that they need. Choosing food that is processed, packed with sugars and fats or artificial ingredients is a sure-fire way to become malnourished over time.

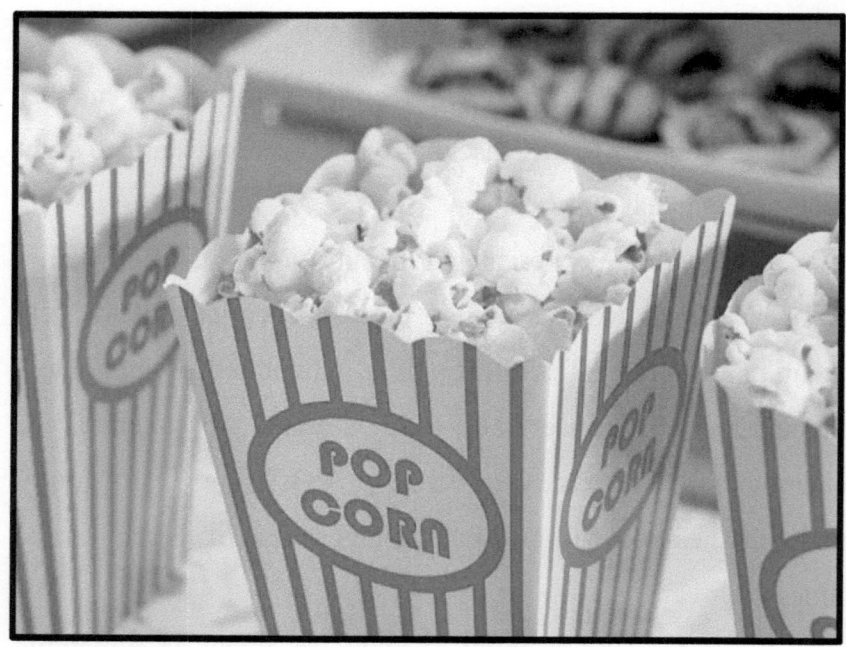

You may believe that you couldn't possibly be suffering from malnutrition because you're eating three meals a day, but if the content of those three meals aren't well-balanced and don't contain the right components, you may as well be starving yourself.

Micronutrient Deficiencies

The human body requires both macronutrients and micronutrients to achieve optimal health and well-being. As you might guess from their name, macronutrients need to be consumed in larger amounts than micronutrients. The human body only requires a small amount of micronutrients to function well.

These minerals and vitamins only need to be consumed in tiny volumes. However, if you don't get those small amounts, you are at a much greater risk of disease, and your immune system will certainly feel the negative impact. Therefore, it's essential to make sure that you're choosing foods that contain plenty of the essential minerals, vitamins and micronutrients to stay fit and healthy and to keep your immunity at the optimal level.

There are close to 30 minerals and vitamins that cannot be manufactured by the body in sufficient amounts. These are known as essential micronutrients. If you don't eat enough foods that contain key minerals, vitamins and other compounds, you are at a higher risk of some major illnesses like cancer, type II diabetes, osteoporosis and heart disease.

The best way of ensuring you're getting enough micronutrients is to eat a well-balanced diet that contains lots of legumes, vegetables, fruits, wholegrains and lean protein sources together with healthy fats like olive oil and nuts.

There are five essential micronutrients that have key roles to play in maintaining your immunity. These are vitamin C, vitamin C6, vitamin E, zinc and magnesium. They can be added to your diet in many ways:

- **Vitamin B6** – eat more chicken, bananas, cereals, potatoes with the skin on and pork loin

- **Vitamin C** – eat citrus fruits, tomatoes, kiwi fruits, broccoli, and sweet peppers

- **Vitamin E** – eat sunflower oil and seeds, safflower oil, almonds, and peanut butter

- **Magnesium** – eat seeds, nuts, legumes, and whole wheat

- **Zinc** – eat beef shank, dark turkey meat and oysters

An Overview of Superfoods

In recent years, you may have heard about superfoods in the media. These foods are touted as the newest and best thing when it comes to keeping yourself in optimal condition. You can keep your body healthy and energized by eating superfoods that are known to improve your immunity, but what are these superfoods, and what do they do to help boost your overall health and well-being?

Superfoods are foods that are known to contain an especially high amount of minerals, antioxidants, and vitamins. With such a high nutrient concentration, this makes them ideal for improving your immunity. The components that they contain all work together to give your immune system valuable assistance so that it can function at the highest possible level.

Some of the superfoods that are known to boost your immune system include:

- Garlic
- Ginger
- Goji berries
- Chia seeds
- Matcha

- ❑ Kale
- ❑ Blueberries

Of course, these aren't the only superfoods out there, but they are among the ones that have been shown in scientific research to have a positive impact on your overall health, well-being and immunity.

By adding some or all of the above foods into your daily diet, it's possible to give your immune system a little extra assistance to do its job and to combat the invading threats that it encounters in the form of bacteria and viruses every day. With this additional power, it can keep you healthier for longer, and make sure that you don't succumb to illnesses that could make you unwell either in the short or long term.

CHAPTER 3

PHYTOCHEMICALS AND IMMUNITY

Phytochemicals have been shown to have an important impact on your immune function and overall well-being. However, many people are unaware that they exist. Unlike superfoods, antioxidants and other well-publicized health-promoting foods, phytochemicals have received little attention from the media. Therefore, they are often overlooked, even by those who are eager to give their health a much-needed boost.

In fact, phytochemicals have been researched for decades, but it's only recently that they've been studied in humans. Yet, findings have shown that these naturally-0ccurring plant chemicals could have a major positive effect on your well-being and immunity. So, it's definitely worth finding out more about them and how you can add them to you daily diet. This will promote your immune system's function and help it to keep you protected from harm.

What are Phytochemicals?

Phytochemicals are plant chemicals that occur naturally and, when consumed, have been shown to interact with the immune system on every level and support it effectively. Phytochemicals have even been shown to inhibit cancer at each stage of its development, stopping new cancer cells from forming, inhibiting their growth, and removing the toxins that can cause cancer.

They can even influence the gene activity that is involved in the development of cancer and suppress the hormones that have been shown to stimulate the growth of certain types of cancer. With this in mind, it's important to be aware of the most beneficial phytochemicals that you could be adding to your daily intake.

The Most Beneficial Phytochemicals

There are several types of phytochemicals that have been shown to be highly beneficial for your immunity. These bioactive chemicals have been proven to slow down and halt cancer progression by inhibiting cell division, altering gene expression, reducing inflammation and free radical damage, and inhibiting the blood supply to tumors.

Quercetin is one frequently studied flavonoid. It can be found in green tea. It blocks the production of hormone receptors, growth factors and the other components known to promote cancer growth. Some other foods that contain phytochemicals that can be beneficial for your immune system include avocados, cranberries and pomegranates.

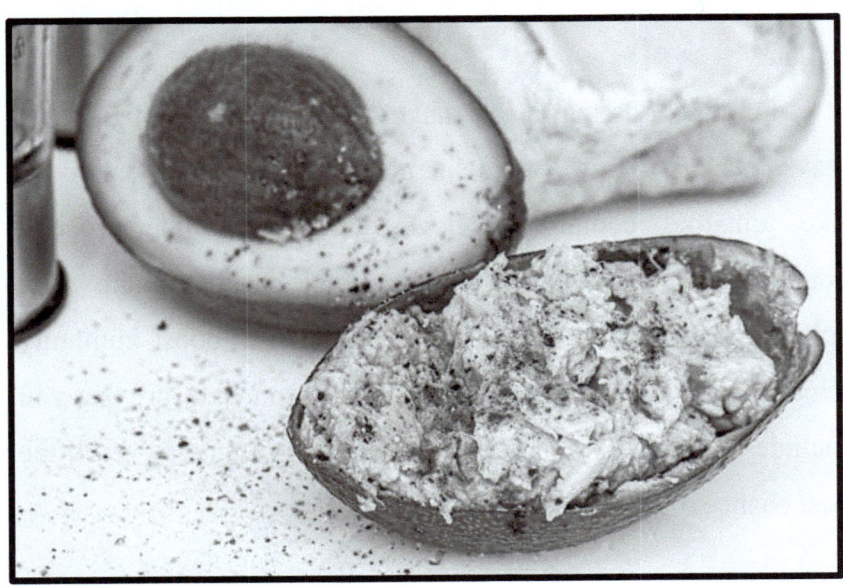

Cranberries contain a number of phytochemicals including polyphenols, flavanol glycosides, proanthocyanidins, phenolic acids and anthocyanins. These compounds can reduce the load on your immune system, helping to keep you safe from illnesses.

Meanwhile, avocados are a rich source of carotenoids and pomegranates are packed with ellagic acid and hydrolysable ellagitannins, both of which are polyphenols.

Black tea and garlic have also been shown to be beneficial phytochemicals. Garlic contains organoselenium metabolites while black tea contains polyphenols like epigallocatechin-3-gallate.

Eating foods that are a range of colors is one of the best ways to benefit from phytochemicals in your diet. Red foods like tomatoes contain lycopene, green food like broccoli contains glucosinolates, and onion and garlic contain allyl sulfides. All of these compounds are known to boost immunity exponentially, so you should try every day to make sure that you include foods of several colors in your meals to give yourself the best chance of achieving optimal immunity.

CHAPTER 4

ANTIOXIDANTS AND IMMUNE HEALTH

Antioxidants have recently been shown to have a powerful part to play in improving your immunity and overall well-being. There has been a lot of news in the media over the last few years touting antioxidants as the biggest and best thing to include in your diet to ensure optimal health. But what are they, and how do they work?

What are Antioxidants?

Antioxidants are substances that are known to slow down or even prevent the damage caused to the body's cells by free radicals – the unstable molecules produced by the body in reaction to environmental factors and other stresses.

Antioxidants can come from either artificial or natural sources. Some plant-based foods are believed to be packed with antioxidants, and plant-based antioxidants are a form of phytonutrient.

Some antioxidants are produced by the body itself. These are known as endogenous antioxidants. Those that are derived from outside your body are called exogenous antioxidants. Antioxidants are known to protect against oxidative stress – the cell damage caused by free radicals in the body.

Some of the processes and activities that can cause oxidative stress include:

Excessive exercise

Mitochondrial activity

Ischemia and reperfusion damage

Tissue trauma because of injury or inflammation

Smoking

Consuming processed and refined foods, artificial sweeteners, trans fats and certain additives and dyes

Environmental pollution

Exposure to drugs, pesticides and chemicals

Radiation

Ozone

Industrial solvents

When cell damage occurs, the result can be:

Excess release of free copper or iron ions

Activation of phagocytes, one of the white blood cell types that combat infection

Disruption in the electron transport chains

Increased enzymes that generate more free radicals

These all cause oxidative stress.

Oxidative stress is linked to vision loss, atherosclerosis, and cancer due to cell changes caused by free radicals. Consuming more antioxidants can reduce these risks.

The Role of Free Radicals

Free radicals are waste substances created by cells when the body reacts to its environment and processes food. When your body can't remove the free radicals efficiently, the result can be oxidative stress which harms the cells and impairs the function of your body.

Oxidative stress caused by free radicals is linked with a host of diseases including cancer, heart disease, strokes, arthritis, immune deficiency, respiratory diseases, Parkinson's disease, emphysema, and other ischemic and inflammatory conditions. When you consume enough antioxidants, the free radicals are neutralized, boosting your overall health.

Which Foods Contain Antioxidants?

It's believed there are hundreds or even thousands of antioxidants. Each one has its own role to play and interacts with others inside the body to keep it functioning properly. Some examples of antioxidants include:

Vitamin A

Vitamin C

Vitamin E

Beta-Carotene

Lutein

Lycopene

Selenium

Zeaxanthin

Manganese

Flavonoids, catechins, flavones, phytoestrogens and polyphenols are all forms of antioxidants found in plant-based food.

All antioxidants serve their own function and cannot be interchanged with others. This is why you need to eat a varied and balanced diet.

Some foods that are known to be rich sources of antioxidants include:

Vitamin A – liver, eggs, and dairy products

Vitamin C – vegetables and fruits including bell peppers, oranges, and berries

Vitamin E – seeds and nuts, vegetable and sunflower oils, and leafy green vegetables

Beta-carotene – vegetables and fruits in bright colors like peas, mangos, carrots, and spinach

Lycopene – red and pink vegetables and fruits like watermelon and tomatoes

Lutein – leafy green vegetables, oranges, papaya, and corn

Selenium – corn, rice, wheat, nuts, wholegrains, legumes, cheese, and eggs

Other foods said to be good antioxidant sources include:

Legumes like kidney beans and black beans

Eggplants

Black and green teas

Red grapes

Pomegranates

Dark chocolate

Goji berries

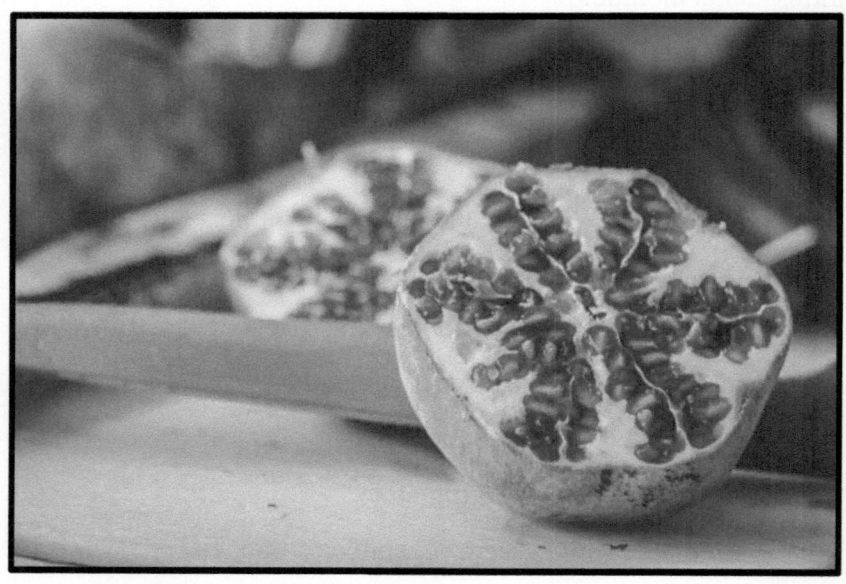

It's important to note that cooking certain foods may decrease or increase their level of antioxidants. For example, when tomatoes are cooked the lycopene inside them becomes easier for the body to use and process. Conversely, zucchini, peas and cauliflower all lose some of their antioxidant potency when they're cooked.

CHAPTER 5

POLYSACCHARIDES –
IMPROVING YOUR WELLBEING

While we're looking at nutrition and how it benefits your immune system, it's impossible to overlook the importance of polysaccharides in your diet. You may never have heard this term used before. However, you can be certain that you will have included polysaccharides in your diet.

What Are Polysaccharides?

Polysaccharides are vital for proper nutrition since they contain complex carbohydrates that are essential energy sources for the body. All bodily functions rely on carbohydrates to produce energy, and although the body is capable of producing some energy itself, it cannot produce enough to make it self-sustainable.

Failing to consume enough carbohydrates means that energy needs to be supplemented by other sources. Insufficient carbohydrates in your diet puts you at risk of physical symptoms such as blood sugar drops, along with feelings of lightheadedness and weakness. Polysaccharides help you to overcome tiredness while supporting healthy blood sugar levels and blood pressure, supporting your immune function, promoting good cardiovascular health, and even boosting your libido!

The Most Common Polysaccharides

Commonly, polysaccharides are found in cereal grain husks, certain yeasts, algae, mushrooms and fungi, and plants. Some common polysaccharides include:

Astragalus root – this polysaccharide is known to stimulate the immune system by increasing stem cell numbers in the lymphatic tissue and spinal cord and encouraging them to turn into immune cells, promoting T lymphocyte activation, stimulating macrophages and immunoglobulin production, stimulating the endogenous production of interferon and inhibiting virus replication.

Laminaria Japonica – this polysaccharide binds strongly with toxic molecules like heavy metals, encouraging them to be eliminated from your body before their harmful effects can be experienced.

Cordyceps Sinensis – rich in polysaccharides, adenosine and cordycepic acid, this mushroom stimulates the immune system.

Goji berries – these contain polysaccharides that powerfully support the body's defense systems by increasing lymphocyte and NK cell activity.

Larchwood – this contains polysaccharides known as arabinogalactans that increase the body's immune system response to disease by stimulating the body's natural killer cells' cytotoxicity and acting on inflammation.

How can I add Polysaccharides into my Diet?

It isn't difficult to add polysaccharides into your daily diet.

Starch is a main example of polysaccharides – the primary carbohydrate source for tubers, plant seeds and vegetables which grow under the ground. Food sources of starch are often called starchy carbohydrates, and include foods such as rice, potatoes and corn as well as pasta, cereal and bread. These foods usually make up the most common type of carbohydrates in your everyday diet. Starches are broken down in the body into glucose, and this supplies the essential energy you need.

Cellulose is another polysaccharide that is found in many foods. It provides a protective structure or covering for vegetables, fruits and seeds. It is cellulose that gives foods their crunchy texture and it cannot be digested by the body. It functions as a dietary fiber source, adding bulk to stools and helping in the maintenance of proper digestive processes. Pear and apple skins contain cellulose, as do wholegrains such as wheat bran and plant leaves such as spinach.

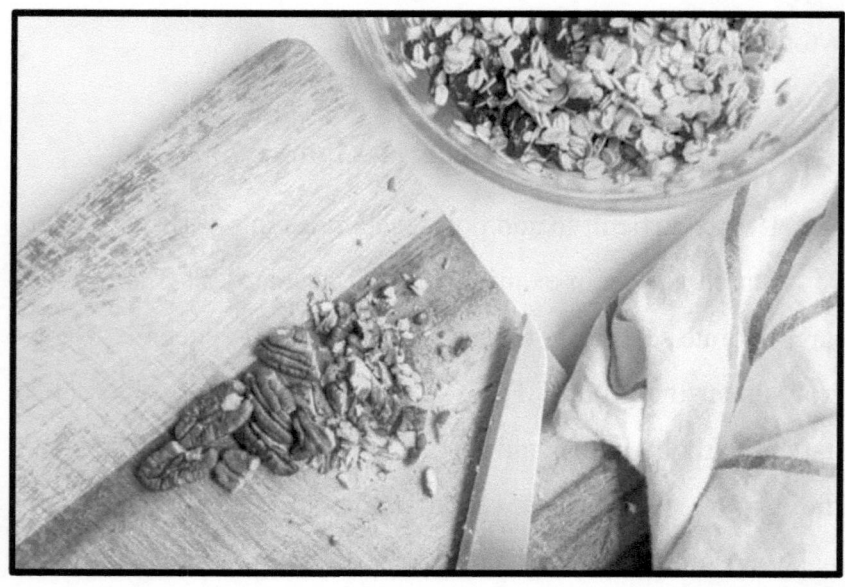

Pectin is another polysaccharide compound which forms a gel - like substance when the body breaks it down. Foods containing pectin are sometimes called soluble fiber sources, and they benefit your body by prolonging the time taken to empty the stomach, helping you feel fuller for longer. Some soluble fiber sources include dried beans, oats, flax seed, barley, nuts, apples, oranges, psyllium husk and carrots.

While starchy foods often have a bad reputation as food sources that are high in fat, they actually contain less than 50 percent of the calories of fat in your diet. Starchy foods are also good sources of iron, calcium, vitamins, and fiber. To maximize their benefits, prepare them in healthy oils such as vegetable or olive oil, and avoid using high-fat methods of preparation such as frying, since this can offset their nutritional value.

CHAPTER 6

PLANT FOODS AND THEIR CANCER
FIGHTING PROPERTIES

A strong link has been found between the development of cancer and a weakened immune system, so it's imperative to find ways of boosting immunity to aid the fight against this life-threatening disease. One way to achieve this is by including more plant foods in your diet.

Cancer and the Immune System

There are specific cancers that directly affect the immune system such as leukemia and lymphoma. However, all kinds of cancer impact immunity.

Cancer cells are created from the body's own cells, and therefore, the immune system sometimes fails to recognize that it needs to attack them. While sometimes our immune systems know the cancer cells are foreign bodies that must be eradicated, more often than not, these cells go unnoticed. In some cases, cancer cells may even switch off the body's immune response making sure immune cells cannot attack them.

Not only that, but cancer sufferers also often have a weak immune system. This happens when cancer itself, or the treatments given to combat the disease, affect the bone marrow. The blood cells are produced inside the bone marrow, so when it's impacted by cancer, radiation or chemotherapy, it produces fewer blood cells than usual. If the blood cell count is low, your body cannot fight off infections properly.

Plant Foods and Their Role in Combating Cancer

There has been some evidence to suggest vegetarians are better able to resist cancer, and it's believed that this happens because plant-based foods like vegetables, fruits, nuts, legumes and wholegrains contain plenty of nutrients. Eating plenty of these types of foods reduces your risk of developing cancer.

This is because plants produce plant chemicals called phytochemicals that can protect the cells from being damaged. Not only that, but plant-based foods increase the amount of fiber we consume, and this also reduces the risk of certain cancers.

Finally, plant-based diets are, in general, lower in calories, and this helps us to maintain a healthy bodyweight which, again, reduces the risk of developing cancer.

This is all paired with the fact that meat may increase the risk of cancer. An extra 3.5 oz of red meat each day increases the risk of developing polyps in the colon by up to 2 percent, and just 1.25 oz of processed meat each day increases this risk by a massive 29 percent.

Which Plant Foods Should I Include in my Diet?

A plant-based diet emphasizes the consumption of minimally processed, wholefoods while limiting or avoiding animal products. The focus is on plants like fruits, vegetables, wholegrains, seeds, nuts and legumes, while refined foods such as white flour, processed oils and added sugars are excluded.

Some of the foods you should add to your daily diet include:

> Fruits such as citrus fruits, berries, peaches, pears, bananas, and pineapple

Vegetables like kale, spinach, broccoli, tomatoes, carrots, cauliflower, peppers, and asparagus

Starchy vegetables such as sweet potatoes, potatoes, and butternut squash

Wholegrains like brown rice, farro, rolled oats, quinoa, pasta, barley, and brown rice

Healthy fats like olive oil, avocados, coconut oil and unsweetened coconut oil

Legumes like peas, lentils, chickpeas, black beans, and peanuts

Nuts, seeds and nut butters like cashews, almonds, pumpkin seeds, macadamia nuts, tahini, and natural peanut butter

Unsweetened plant-based milk like almond, cashew, or coconut milks

Herbs, spices and seasonings like rosemary, basil, curry, turmeric, salt, and black pepper

Condiments like mustard, salsa, soy sauce, lemon juice, vinegar, and nutritional yeast

Plant-based proteins like tempeh and tofu

Beverages like tea, coffee, and water

Certain foods should also be avoided. These include:

Fast food

Added sweets and sugars

Refined grains

Convenience and packaged foods

Processed vegan foods

Artificial sweeteners

Processed animal products

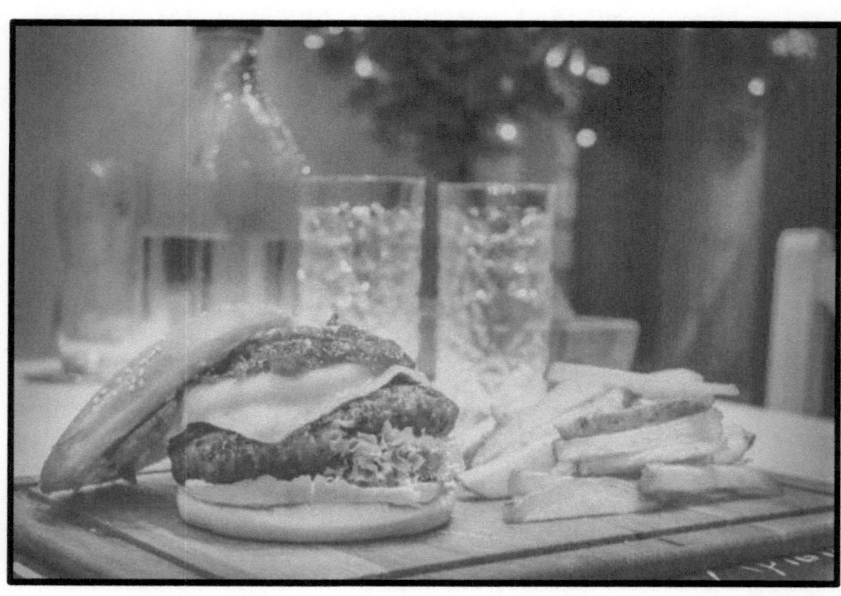

CHAPTER 7

OMEGA-3 HELPS TO FIGHT DISEASE

Boosting your immunity to combat disease can be achieved by adding Omega-3 fatty acids to your diet. You may have heard of these fatty acids in terms of fish oils and supplements, but it's possible to add them into your diet through natural food sources too.

What is Omega-3?

Omega-3s are types of essential fatty acids which have a key role to play in the human body and which offer several health benefits. Since they cannot be produced by the body itself, they have to be derived from your daily diet.

There are three key types of Omega-3s. These are:

ALA – Alpha Linolenic Acid

DHA – Docosahexaenoic Acid

EPA – Eicosapentaenoic Acid

While the first of these is primarily found in plant-based foods, EPA and DHA are mostly found in algae and animal products.

Some common foods that have a high level of Omega-3s include fish oils, fatty fish, chia seeds, flax seeds, walnuts, and flaxseed oil.

Neutralizing Inflammation

Whenever you think of the word "inflammation" you're probably thinking about pain, and, in many ways, this is the case. Inflammation's purpose is primarily to protect the place where an injury or illness has occurred. It encourages the body's immune system to heal and repair damaged tissues. However, when inflammation is allowed to continue unabated, it throws biological functions out of alignment.

Usually, chronic inflammation is a painless condition and is characterized by damage from free radicals. It isn't linked to a specific tissue, so could trigger all types of condition from autoimmune diseases to allergic reactions.

Nutrition has a pivotal role when it comes to fighting and preventing inflammation. There are several foods that are known to promote inflammation, including fatty meats, white bread, processed cheese and vegetable oils, but eating more anti-inflammatory foods supports the body's own defenses against the damage caused by free radicals.

There is plenty of scientific evidence to suggest that the Omega-3s that are found in oily fish helps to combat inflammation inside the body. Eating two or three portions of mackerel, sardines, tuna or herring each week may help you to combat disease and boost your immunity.

Good Dietary Sources of Omega-3

Omega-3 fatty acids can be found occurring naturally in certain foods and may also be added to fortified foods. It's possible to get plenty of Omega-3 in your diet by including these foods in your regime:

Fish and seafood, particularly salmon, tuna, mackerel, sardines, and herring

Seeds and nuts like walnuts, chia seeds and flaxseed

Plant oils like canola, soybean, and flaxseed oils

Fortified food like certain brands of yogurt, eggs, milk, juice, and soy beverages.

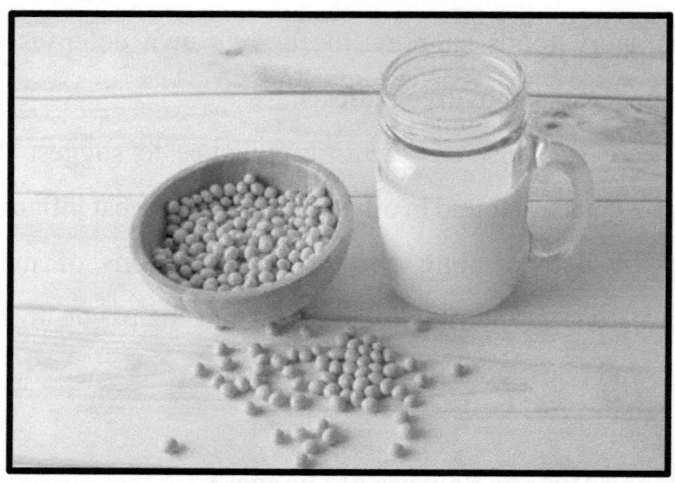

CHAPTER 8

PREBIOTICS AND YOUR IMMUNITY

When it comes to your immunity, the gut has been found to have an important part to play. Maintaining good gut health can give your body's immune system a boost, and prebiotics have a role to play in this.

The Role of the gut in Immunity

Most of us know that keeping our gut healthy is important, and this involves maintaining a healthy gut microbiota.

Researchers have discovered and recognized that the body's other organ systems can be influenced by the gut environment and it's now becoming realized that poor gut health could cause many diseases and conditions like lung disease or depression.

Our immune systems form the primary link between the gut bacteria and the way in which they influence our well-being. At one time it was believed that the uterus was bacteria-free, however, it's now been found that bacteria can be detected in the placenta, ensuring that babies are exposed to bacteria from before birth. We're all born with an underdeveloped immune system and therefore rely on the antibodies provided by our mothers at first, but our immune cells then learn the best ways of protecting our bodies from illnesses once all the material antibodies have worn away. Bacteria in the gut is essential in this education process.

Research has shown that gut bacteria maintains balance in our immune systems. During our lives, we're exposed continually to new things inside the gut, the lungs and the nose through our environment and the food that we consume. Things like food additives, the non-pathogenic microorganisms found in dirt or dust, and pollen in the air we breathe all enter our bodies. Luckily, when our immune systems are healthy, they can handle these invaders easily.

For those with an impaired immune system, inflammatory responses are triggered each time a new food is tried or each time a new substance is encountered. The immune system is required to maintain the right balance between tolerance and reaction. This tolerance is known as oral tolerance. It can be established by maintaining diverse gut flora with lots of different fungi, microorganisms and bacteria to teach the immune system's cells which invaders are bad and which can be safely overlooked.

The bacterial balance in the gut influences our immune system's balance. If the balance is off, the immune system may adopt an increased inflammatory state that goes on to affect the other systems in the body, increasing the chances of developing a range of diseases including Type I and II diabetes, depression and obesity.

Although most bacteria are beneficial, there are some that cause diseases to progress. Bacteria also adjusts to its current environment. This means that, when good bacteria become removed because of medication or dietary changes, some opportunistic pathogens move in to fill up the gap that remains. This, of course, leads to further problems, more inflammation and health concerns.

It isn't easy to permanently change the gut flora once it has been established. Once it has been disturbed, it usually returns to its normal state in a short space of time. So, for example, if you go abroad on vacation and eat different foods, your gut will return to normal on your return home.

However, imbalanced gut flora can loop in negative cycles, reinforcing harmful functions. It is a lack of bacterial diversity that causes a skewed microbiota – maintaining diversity means that your gut can bounce back more rapidly from any unhealthy dietary fluctuations and is more capable of withstanding outside intruders. As a result, your immune system will be better-regulated and considerably more tolerant of change. As a result, you will be more resistant to disease and illnesses.

What are Prebiotics and how can They Help?

Prebiotics are food components that are known to improve the supply of food for the microorganisms that live inside our gastrointestinal tracts. They are capable of giving the beneficial bacteria in our guts the nourishment they need and, therefore, the best possible chance of growing and flourishing. It's possible to boost the level of prebiotics in your body naturally by eating more vegetables and fruits.

How can Prebiotics be Added to the Diet?

There are a number of foods that are known to be beneficial prebiotics. These include:

Chicory root – popular thanks to its coffee-like taste, chicory root is a valuable source of prebiotics. Almost half of the fiber in chicory root comes from inulin, a prebiotic fiber. This nourishes the bacteria in the gut, improves your digestion and relieves your constipation. It also helps to boost the production of bile in the body which, in turn, improves the digestion of fat. Not only that, but chicory root contains a lot of antioxidant compounds known to protect your liver from oxidative damage.

Dandelion greens – these greens are ideal for inclusion in a salad and they are an excellent source of fiber, containing as much as 4g of fiber in each 100g serving. Much of that fiber is derived from inulin which reduces constipation, increases the amount of good bacteria in your gut and boosts your immune system. Dandelion greens have diuretic, antioxidant, anti- inflammatory, cholesterol-lowering, and anti-cancer effects that can help you to stay healthy and well.

Jerusalem artichokes – sometimes called the Earth Apple, the Jerusalem artichoke offers a host of health benefits. It supplies around 2g of dietary fiber in every 100g and 76 percent of this fiber is derived from inulin. This food increases the good bacteria in your good, strengthens your immune system and even prevents specific metabolic disorders. Not only that, but it is high in potassium and thiamine, both of which aid the nervous system, promoting good muscle function.

Garlic – this tasty herb has been linked with many health benefits. Around 11 percent of its fiber content is derived from inulin, with 6 percent coming from a naturally occurring sweet probiotic known as fructooligosaccharides. Garlic is a prebiotic that promotes Bifidobacteria growth inside the gut. These beneficial bacteria also help to prevent disease-promoting bacteria from growing. Garlic also reduces the chance of developing heart disease thanks to its antimicrobial, anti-cancer and antioxidant effects.

Onions – these vegetables are versatile and tasty, but they also offer a host of health benefits, with inulin accounting for 10 percent of their fiber content and fructooligosaccharides making up another 6 percent.

As a result, the gut flora is strengthened while fat breakdown is aided, and the immune system boosted by increasing the production of nitric oxide in the cells. Furthermore, onions have a high level of quercetin, the flavonoid that gives this vegetable its anti-cancer and antioxidant properties.

Leeks – coming from the same vegetable family as garlic and onions, leeks offer similar benefits for your health. They contain as much as 16 percent inulin fiber and this helps to promote the growth of healthy bacteria in the gut while also helping to break down fat. Also, leeks have a high amount of flavonoids which help to support the body's natural response to oxidative stress.

Asparagus – this popular vegetable represents another excellent prebiotic source, with around 2 to 3 grams of inulin content in every 100-gram serving. Asparagus promotes the growth of friendly bacteria inside the gut and is associated with the prevention of some cancers. By combining antioxidants and fiber, asparagus offers anti-inflammatory benefits.

Bananas – these popular fruits are rich in fiber, minerals and vitamins while also containing a small amount of inulin. Unripe bananas contain large amounts of resistant starch and this has a prebiotic effect that increases the number of healthy bacteria in the gut while reducing bloating.

Barley – this cereal grain contains 3 to 8 grams of beta-glucan in every 100-gram serving. This prebiotic fiber promotes friendly bacteria growth inside your digestive tract. It also lowers your LDL and total cholesterol and blood sugar while also being rich in selenium to boost thyroid function, provides antioxidant benefits and improves immunity.

Oats – healthy whole oat is a grain with prebiotic benefits. Oats contain a large amount of beta-glucan fiber together with some resistant starch. The beta-glucan found in oats is associated with healthier gut bacteria as well as improved blood sugar control, lower levels of

LDL cholesterol and a reduced risk of cancer. Oats also offer anti-inflammatory and antioxidant protection for the body thanks to the phenolic acid they contain.

Apples – not only are apples delicious but pectin makes up around half of the total fiber content of an apple. As we've already pointed out, pectin offers benefits to your immune system. Its prebiotic advantages include its ability to increase butyrate – the short-chain fatty acid which feeds good bacteria in the gut while decreasing the number of bad bacteria.

Apples also contain a high level of polyphenol antioxidants, and when pectin and polyphenols are combined, fat metabolism and digestive health are improved. Not only that, but apples have anti-inflammatory and antioxidant properties that help to reduce the chances of developing illnesses and diseases.

Konjac root – sometimes called elephant yam, is a tuber that can sometimes be used as a supplement to offer health benefits. It contains 40 percent glucomannan fiber which is an extremely viscous dietary fiber. Glucomannan fiber in konjac promotes good bacteria growth inside the colon, relieving constipation and boosting your immunity. It also reduces your blood cholesterol levels and helps to promote weight loss while also improving how your body metabolizes carbohydrates.

Cocoa – cocoa beans aren't just delicious, they're also very healthy. When cocoa beans break down inside the colon, nitric oxide is produced, and this offers benefits to your cardiovascular system. Cocoa is one of the best sources of flavanols which has a number of powerful prebiotic benefits, helping to boost the growth of good gut bacteria while benefiting your heart health.

Burdock Root – popular in Japan, burdock root offers many health benefits, containing around 4 grams of fiber in every 100-gram serving, with most of this fiber being from inulin and FOS. The FOS and inulin in burdock root have prebiotic properties, inhibiting the growth of the bad bacteria in your intestines while improving immune function and promoting healthy bowel movements. Burdock root also offers anti-inflammatory and antioxidant properties while lowering your blood sugar levels.

Flaxseeds – these seeds are very healthy and an excellent source of prebiotics. Containing around 20-40 percent soluble fiber from mucilage gums and 60-80 percent insoluble fiber from lignin and cellulose, the fiber found in flaxseeds boosts the number of good bacteria in your gut, promoting healthy bowel movements and reducing the amount of fat in your diet that you absorb and digest. Also, since flaxseeds contain phenolic antioxidants, they offer antioxidant and anti-cancer properties while helping to regulate your blood sugar level.

Yacon root – similar to sweet potato, yacon root is packed with fiber, especially prebiotic FOS (fructooligosaccharides) and inulin. The inulin found in yacon root improves healthy gut bacteria, reducing constipation, enhancing your immunity, improving the absorption of minerals in the body and helping to regulate fats in the blood. Also, yacon root contains phenolic compounds that boost its antioxidant properties.

Jicama root – this root is high in fiber but low in calories. It contains a lot of inulin, a prebiotic fiber that helps to boost your digestive health, enhance your sensitivity to insulin and lower your blood sugar level. It is also in vitamin C that stimulates your immune system to combat diseases.

Wheat bran – this outer layer of whole wheat grain is a great prebiotic source that contains a special kind of fiber made up of AXOS (arabinoxylan oligosaccharides). AXOS fiber makes up as much as 64-69 percent of the fiber content of wheat bran and allows it to boost the levels of good Bifidobacteria inside the gut. Not only that, but wheat bran reduces digestive problems like abdominal pain, cramping and flatulence. Grains that are rich in AXOS also offer anti-cancer and antioxidant properties.

Seaweed – although seaweed isn't eaten often, it's a powerful prebiotic to add to your diet. Around 50 to 85 percent of the fiber content of seaweed is derived from the water-soluble fiber. This enhances good gut bacteria growth while preventing bad bacteria from growing. It also boosts your immune function, reducing your chances of developing colon cancer. Also, seaweed is rich in the antioxidants that have been associated with strokes and heart attack prevention.

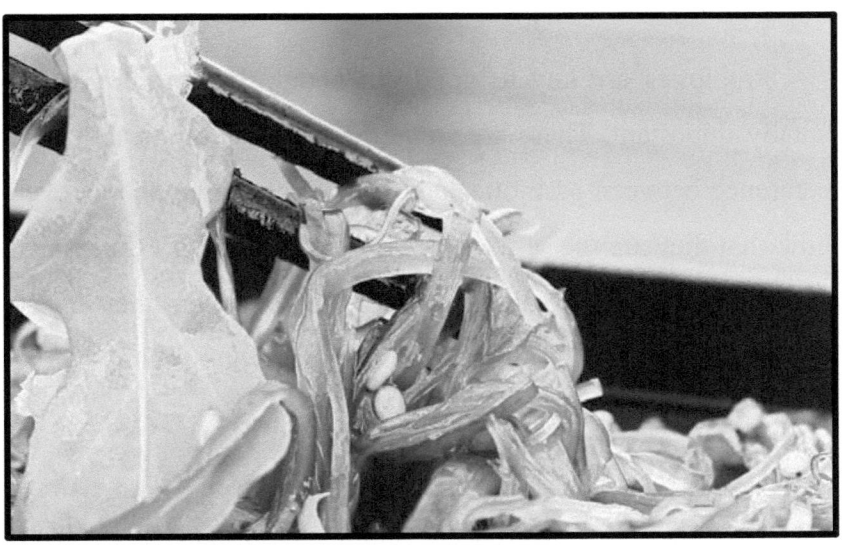

CHAPTER 9

PROBIOTICS AND THE GUT

Prebiotics are key to good gut health, but probiotics are equally important. There are some misunderstandings about the difference between prebiotics and probiotics. Some people even think that they are the same thing. However, this isn't the case at all. Probiotics are very different from prebiotics, but they are no less vital to good gut health and a strong immune system.

What Are Probiotics?

Probiotics are live yeasts and bacteria that offer many health benefits, especially for the digestive system. Usually, we think of bacteria as being bad for you and causing diseases. However, the human body is actually full of different bacteria. While some bacteria are bad, others are good and can help to keep the gut healthy and functioning properly.

Probiotics can be found in certain foods such as yogurt as well as in certain supplements. They are often recommended by doctors to aid in the relief of digestive disturbances.

Probiotics work to keep us healthy by:

Replacing the good bacteria inside the body that are lost through taking antibiotics.

Balancing the bad and good bacteria levels so your body can continue to function in the way that it should.

Many bacterial types are kinds of probiotic. All offer different benefits. However, the majority are covered by two main groups:

Lactobacillus – this probiotic is the most common. You find it in fermented foods and yogurt. Different strains help to treat diarrhea and may be helpful for people who are unable to digest the sugar in milk known as lactose.

Bifidobacterium – this probiotic can also be found in some types of dairy product. It helps to reduce the symptoms associated with IBS (irritable bowel syndrome) and some other conditions.

Saccharomyces Boulardii is a yeast that can be found in probiotics. It helps combat digestive problems and diarrhea.

How can Probiotics Improve Immunity?

It's known that probiotics can boost your immune system, inhibiting harmful gut bacterial growth in your body. Not only that, but some probiotics promote your body's natural antibody production. They may even boost the immune cells such as T lymphocytes, natural killer cells and IgA-producing cells.

Reviews have found that if you take probiotics, you're less likely to suffer from respiratory infections, and any you do develop will last for less time. The probiotic known as Lactobacillus Crispatus has also been proven to reduce the chances of developing a urinary tract infection by as much as 50 percent.

How can I Include More Probiotics in my Diet?

Although there are a number of different types and classes of probiotics, some common ones include:

Lactobacillus

Bifidobacterium

Saccharomyces Boulardii

Sometimes, food manufacturers call probiotics "active cultures" or "live cultures". They are all the same thing. Many fermented foods contain probiotics. This essentially means that the bacteria inside those foods are still alive. Often, the process of producing food destroys any living bacteria in them. When products are left on a store shelf without being refrigerated, it may be unable to contain active and live probiotics.

Some dairy products that are known to contain probiotics include:

Kefir (a probiotic milk drink)

Aged cheeses like mozzarella, gouda, and cheddar

Traditional uncultured buttermilk

Yogurts

However, there are some foods that aren't dairy but still contain probiotics. These include:

Non-dairy yogurt

Sour, fresh dill pickles

Kombucha (a fermented tea)

Kimchi

Miso

Sauerkraut

Natto (made from fermented soybean)

Water or brine-cured olives

Tempeh

Many different probiotic foods are available, and this means that you have plenty of options when it comes to including them in your daily diet. There is sure to be something to suit your individual tastes, whether you prefer sweet or savory foods.

Some ways of adding probiotics to your healthy diet include:

Having a breakfast made up of probiotic yogurt along with nuts, flax seeds and berries.

Making a stir fry that uses tempeh instead of meat. Make sure to add tempeh right at the end of the cooking process since excessive heat may destroy its active cultures.

Adding miso into soup.

Drinking beverages that are rich in probiotics like kombucha or kefir as a snack in the mid-morning.

Serving sauerkraut alongside your main meal as a side dish.

Remember though that certain foods like yogurt often contain extra sugars, so try to choose ones that contain minimal sugars, artificial sweeteners, and artificial flavorings to ensure the best possible health.

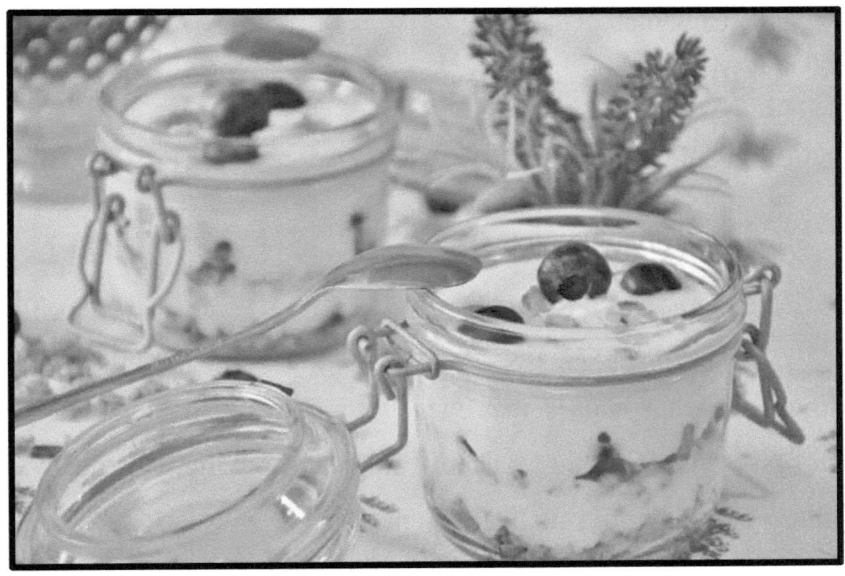

Bear in mind too, that there are some misconceptions about probiotics. Just because certain types of food contain probiotics, that doesn't mean that other similar food types do. As an example, not every yogurt will contain active and live cultures, and those that do will usually be clearly marked.

Also, not every type of fermented food contains live cultures. Some fermented foods that don't contain probiotics include:

> Chocolate
>
> Beer
>
> Wine
>
> Soya sauce
>
> Sourdough bread

That is because these foods have undergone additional processing that causes the live cultures to be made inactive. Processes like filtering, pasteurization and baking kill the live cultures so they offer no health benefits.

CHAPTER 10

TOP 10 IMMUNITY BOOSTING FOODS
TO ADD TO YOUR DIET

Are you ready to experience the benefits that come along with adding immunity boosting foods to your everyday diet? As you've already seen, there are many different ways to increase your immunity simply by changing what you eat each day. So, whether you're ready to add more prebiotics, probiotics, antioxidants or polysaccharides into your eating regime, here are ten of the top foods you should consider eating more of. This will improve your resistance to illnesses and diseases.

1. Citrus Fruits

You've almost certainly been told at some point that vitamin C should be your first port of call if you've caught a cold, and there's a good reason for this. Vitamin C is known to help boost your immune system. It does this by increasing the number of white blood cells that your body produces, and this holds the key to combating infections. Virtually all citrus fruits have a high vitamin C content, and since there are so many different ones to pick from, you can easily add this vitamin into any meal. Some popular citrus fruits are:

Grapefruits

Clementines

Oranges

Tangerines

Limes

Lemons

Since the human body can't store or produce vitamin C you have to eat it every day to continue in good health. Adults are recommended to eat 75 mg each day if they are female or 90 mg each day if they are male.

2. Red Bell Peppers

Citrus fruits contain plenty of vitamin C, but amazingly red bell peppers contain around three times more vitamin C than a Florida orange together with plenty of beta carotene. Vitamin C doesn't just boost your immunity, it also improves the condition of your skin, while beta carotene is converted by the body into vitamin A to promote healthy skin and eyes.

3. Broccoli

Supercharged with minerals and vitamins, broccoli contains lots of vitamins E, C and A together with antioxidants and fiber. This makes it an especially healthy vegetable. To keep it as potent as possible it should be eaten raw or only lightly cooked. Steaming is one of the best ways to preserve its beneficial nutrients.

4. Garlic

Found in virtually every world cuisine, garlic adds zing to your food and also improves your health and well-being. Its value in combating infections has been recognized for generations, and it may also slow down the hardening of the arteries as well as lowering blood pressure. The immune boosting properties of garlic are due to its high concentration of allicin and other sulfur- containing compounds.

5. Ginger

You may have heard about people using ginger if they are sick, and this is due to its anti-inflammatory properties. It can help reduce inflammatory illnesses and sore throats while also helping to combat nausea. When it's incorporated into sweet desserts, it packs heat in the shape of gingerol, which is related to capsaicin. Ginger has also been shown to decrease chronic pain while also possessing cholesterol-lowering properties.

6. Spinach

Not only does spinach have a high vitamin C content, it's also packed with beta carotene and other antioxidants. Both of these can boost your immune system's infection-fighting capabilities. Like broccoli, spinach should be minimally cooked to preserve its nutrients, but if it's cooked lightly, its vitamin A content can be more easily absorbed, and other nutrients can be more easily released from an antinutrient known as oxalic acid.

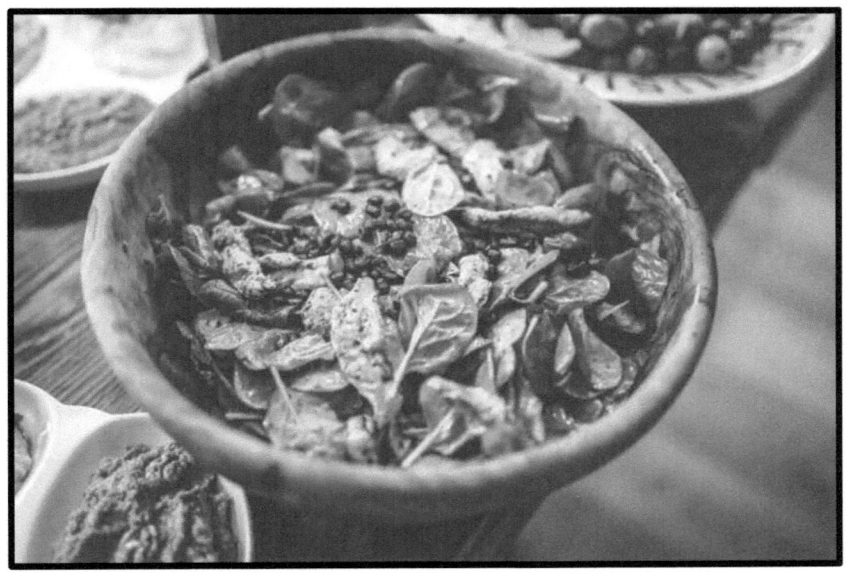

7. Yogurt

You should look out for yogurt that is marked with a phrase saying that it contains active and live cultures. Greek yogurt is one such type. These cultures are believed to stimulate the immune system to fight disease. Whenever possible, choose plain yogurts instead of flavored ones that are packed with sugar.

It's possible to sweeten a plain yogurt yourself using a little honey and some healthy fruit like berries. Yogurt is also a good vitamin D source, so try choosing brands that have been fortified with that vitamin. Vitamin D regulates your immune system, boosting your natural defense against disease.

8. Almonds

When you want to prevent or fight off a cold, you probably choose vitamin C over vitamin E, yet vitamin E is a potent antioxidant that can hold the key to a well-functioning and healthy immune system. Vitamin E is fat-soluble, so it requires fat to be present in order to be properly absorbed.

Nuts like almonds are filled with this vitamin and they also contain healthy fats. An adult only requires around 15 mg of vitamin E daily. Forty-six shelled whole almonds (or a half cup serving) will provide all of your recommended daily intake.

9. Sunflower Seeds

These seeds are packed with nutrients like magnesium, phosphorous, and vitamins E and B6. Vitamin E has a key role to play in maintaining and regulating the function of your immune system. Some other foods that contain a lot of vitamin E include dark leafy greens and avocados. Not only are sunflower seeds high in these nutrients, they also have a high selenium content. Only 1 oz contains 50 percent of the selenium the average adult requires each day.

10. Turmeric

Turmeric is often used in curry and this bitter, bright yellow spice has historically been used as an anti-inflammatory to treat both rheumatoid arthritis and osteoarthritis. A high concentration of curcumin (that gives turmeric its yellow coloring) helps to reduce the damage to the muscles caused by exercise. It also helps to boost the immune system to protect you from illnesses and diseases.

CONCLUSION

Maintaining a healthy immune system couldn't be more important if you want to live a long and healthy life. Without a well-functioning immune system, you are at a high risk of developing an illness or disease.

Once you have become sick, you will struggle to combat it and fight it off to return to full health. From struggling to overcome the common cold to finding it difficult for wounds to heal after an injury, an impaired immune system brings a host of issues that would be better avoided.

It's also important to understand the importance of a strong immune system when it comes to preventing serious health conditions like cancer. Cancer has been linked to a poorly functioning immune system, and if you already have cancer, the treatments that are given to help can reduce the function of the immune system still further.

Chemotherapy and radiation therapy both impact your immunity negatively, putting you at even greater risk of suffering from other illnesses. Therefore, ensuring that you take every step to keep your immunity at optimal level is essential.

As you've seen in this book, one of the best ways to improve your immune system is through a healthy diet. We all know that eating well, with well-balanced meals on a daily basis, can keep us at an appropriate bodyweight. That will ensure that we stay as well as possible. However, we don't always realize the effect that nutrition can have on our immune systems.

If we suffer from malnutrition, our immune system suffers. A lack of micronutrients like vitamins and minerals can lead, in the end, to illnesses, diseases and ongoing medical problems. Therefore, ensuring that you avoid the dangers of malnutrition is imperative to protect your overall well-being.

Not only is it possible to protect your immunity by avoiding malnutrition through eating a well-balanced, healthy diet every day, but you can actively give your immune system a boost by adding certain foods into your dietary regime. There are a number of different food items that have been shown in scientific research to offer a host of benefits for the immune system. These give it a little additional support when it comes to combating diseases and illnesses and eradicating the invaders that it encounters on a daily basis.

Some of the foods that you should be including in your daily diet to improve your immunity include:

Superfoods such as berries, garlic, kale and chia seeds that are known to contain beneficial compounds and nutrients that promote good immune health.

Phytochemicals – plant-derived chemicals that have anti- inflammatory properties to boost the immune system and help it to combat the invaders that it encounters.

Antioxidants – there are many foods that contain antioxidants and that are known to reduce inflammation in the body and combat the free radicals that are responsible for the oxidative stress that causes illnesses of many kinds.

Polysaccharides – these compounds support the body's natural immunity by boosting the effectiveness of the cells' destroying properties.

Plant-based foods – foods that are derived from plants have been shown to help protect you from cancer and other diseases related to the immune system.

Prebiotics – these foods can help to protect the gut through the fiber that they contain and this, in turn, boosts your body's natural immunity.

Probiotics – these foods are known to boost good gut health, reducing the number of bad bacteria and increasing the number of good bacteria. So, you can have a better balance of the essential gut flora that are required to ensure optimal protection against disease and optimal immunity for your body.

The overall message is that eating healthy foods like wholegrains, legumes, healthy oils, fruits, vegetables and fermented foods is the best way to boost your body's own natural immune system. Therefore, you can have the best possible chance of a long and happy life with minimal chance of serious diseases. With a strong immune system, you're less likely to get sick, and if you do, you'll have a good chance of being able to fight off the disease before it causes any serious harm.

Printed by Libri Plureos GmbH in Hamburg, Germany